My Little Brother Is A Trooper

The Story of a Child
With a Dual Diagnosis:

Down Syndrome and Hirschsprung Disease

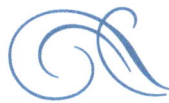

Written and Illustrated by

Isabelle Schnadig

My Little Brother Is a Trooper, Published January, 2025

Editorial and proofreading services: Taylor Morris, Gina Sartirana
Interior layout and cover design: Howard Johnson
Interior and cover illustrations: © Isabelle Schnadig

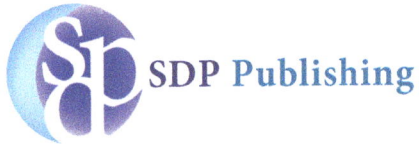

SDP Publishing

Published by SDP Publishing, an imprint of SDP Publishing Solutions, LLC.

To obtain permission(s) to use material from this work, please submit an email request to:
SDP Publishing
Permissions Department
info@SDPPublishing.com.

ISBN-13 (print): 979-8-9885439-7-8
ISBN-13 (ebook): 979-8-9885439-8-5

Printed in the United States of America

THIS BOOK IS DEDICATED TO MY MOST LOVING FAMILY:
MY DEAR HUSBAND ERIC AND OUR FOUR AMAZING
CHILDREN CLAIRE, PAUL, NATHALIE, AND ADRIEN,
WITH MY EVERLASTING LOVE.

ACKNOWLEDGMENTS

When I was pregnant 19 years ago, our baby, Adrien, was diagnosed with Down syndrome. Although we were prepared for Down syndrome, we were totally unprepared for any additional and complex medical conditions. We heard the name "Hirschsprung" for the first time four days after he was born. Adrien's abdomen was swollen, and he was in pain. He had to be rushed from our local hospital to the Neonatal Intensive Care Unit (NICU) at Massachusetts General Hospital (MGH). There, a biopsy confirmed the doctors' diagnosis: there were no nerve cells (ganglia) in his colon. This explained why he could not poop normally: His colon could not relax.

Over the past 18 years, it has been hard to know which of those two conditions has been more impactful in Adrien's developmental delays. Our family has come to say that "HD is always ruling over DS."

I am pleased to publish this children's book with its unique perspective, featuring a kid born with a dual diagnosis under the auspices of REACHirschsprung's Inc. (research, education, and advocacy for children and families with Hirschsprung Disease), a nonprofit committed to "improving the lives of children and families affected by Hirschsprung Disease."

I am grateful to the many people who help both the Hirschsprung and Down syndrome communities meet the challenges of those conditions. Thank you doctors, researchers, other medical professionals, and caregivers! You help heal the sick, discover new treatments, and share best practices to meet the needs of those communities.

Thank you to all the parents and families who care for children with both HD and DS. Those two challenges are immense! It is very impactful to have a community that shares daily challenges, achievements (big and small), pains, and joys.

A special thank you to all the special education teachers who have been so instrumental in helping Adrien learn and become the person he is today.

Thank you also to the REACH board! I am so grateful to each of you.

Finally, thank you to my family and friends for all their support during those challenging years.

About Kids with Down Syndrome and Hirschsprung Disease

According to the National Down Syndrome Society, "The occurrence of having a child with Down syndrome is 1 to every 800 to 1,000 births." About 6,000 babies are born with Down syndrome in the US each year.

Hirschsprung Disease affects approximately 1 in 5,000 births accounting for over 850 new cases yearly in the US and 26,000 worldwide.

"About 2–3% of patients with Down syndrome (DS) have Hirschsprung (HD). Looking at the reverse, of all the patients with HD, about 7% of them have DS."

(*https://pubmed.ncbi.nlm.nih.gov/23943251/*)

DS is the most frequent chromosomal abnormality associated with HD. "The association of HD with DS is well-recognized with an incidence of 7.32%. Many patients with DS continue to have persistent bowel dysfunction after surgical treatment of HD. Our data provides strong evidence that the coexistence of HD and DS is associated with higher rates of pre-/postoperative enterocolitis, poorer functional outcomes, and increased mortality." (Source: "Hirschsprung's disease associated with Down syndrome: a meta-analysis of incidence, functional outcomes and mortality." *Florian Friedmacher, Prem Puri*)

In addition, kids with Down syndrome tend to grow and develop more slowly than other children. They may start walking or talking later than other babies. Special help, such as physical therapy and speech therapy, can give kids a boost with their walking and talking skills. Moreover, many of those children will need more help developing skills such as self-feeding and drinking.

A child with dual diagnoses will likely have complex medical needs, and this will influence his/her overall developmental delays. For instance, toileting may remain an issue for a long time, if not a lifelong endeavor.

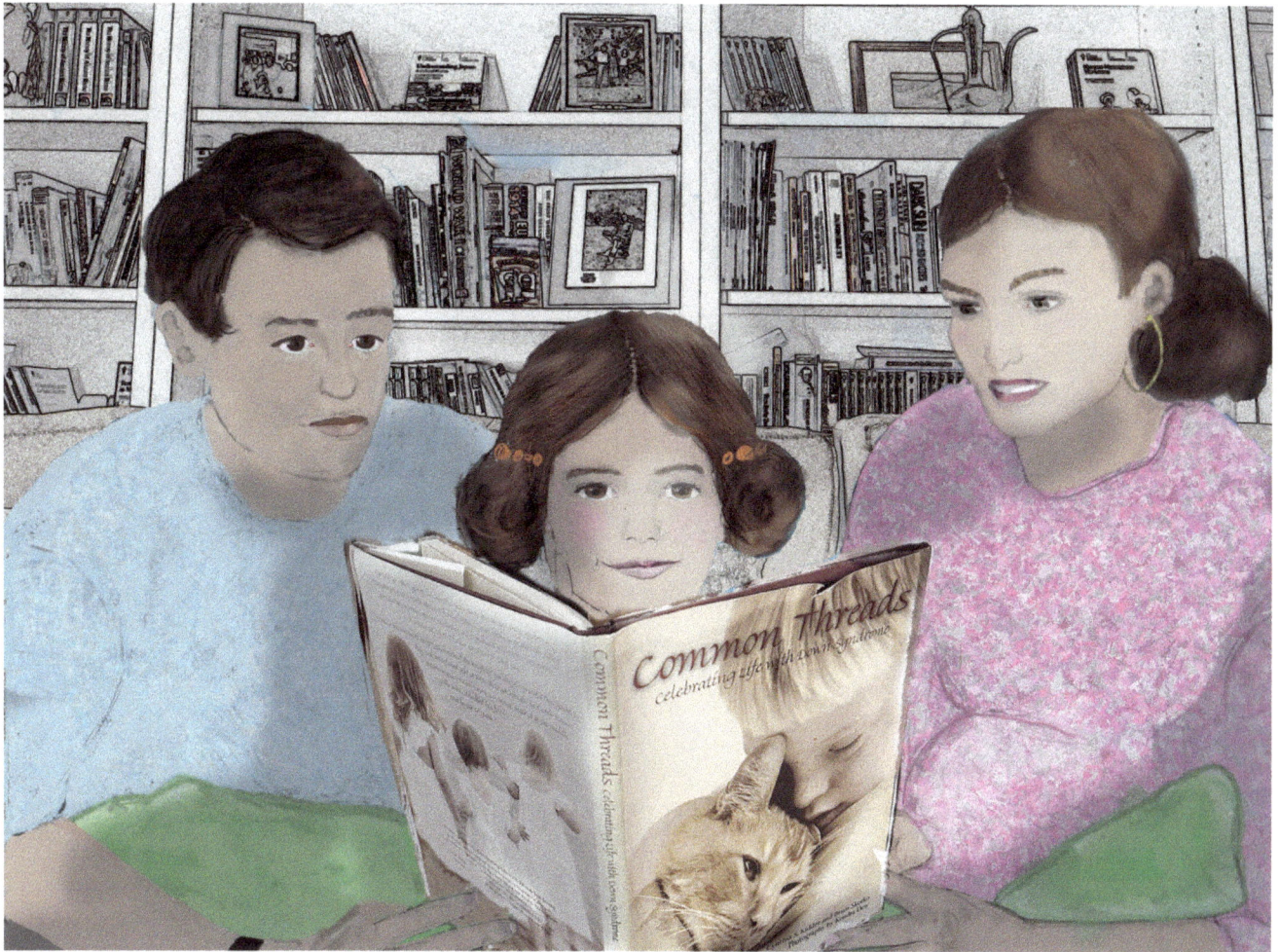

Let me tell you about my little brother Peter, who is a real trooper. My name is Lily, and my brother Peter, who is 16 years old now, grew up facing lots of challenges and struggles.

We knew before Peter was born that he had **Down syndrome**. Mom had an ultrasound early in her pregnancy. The doctor told us then that my little brother had an extra **chromosome** which made him very special; he will make us smile and always surprise us.

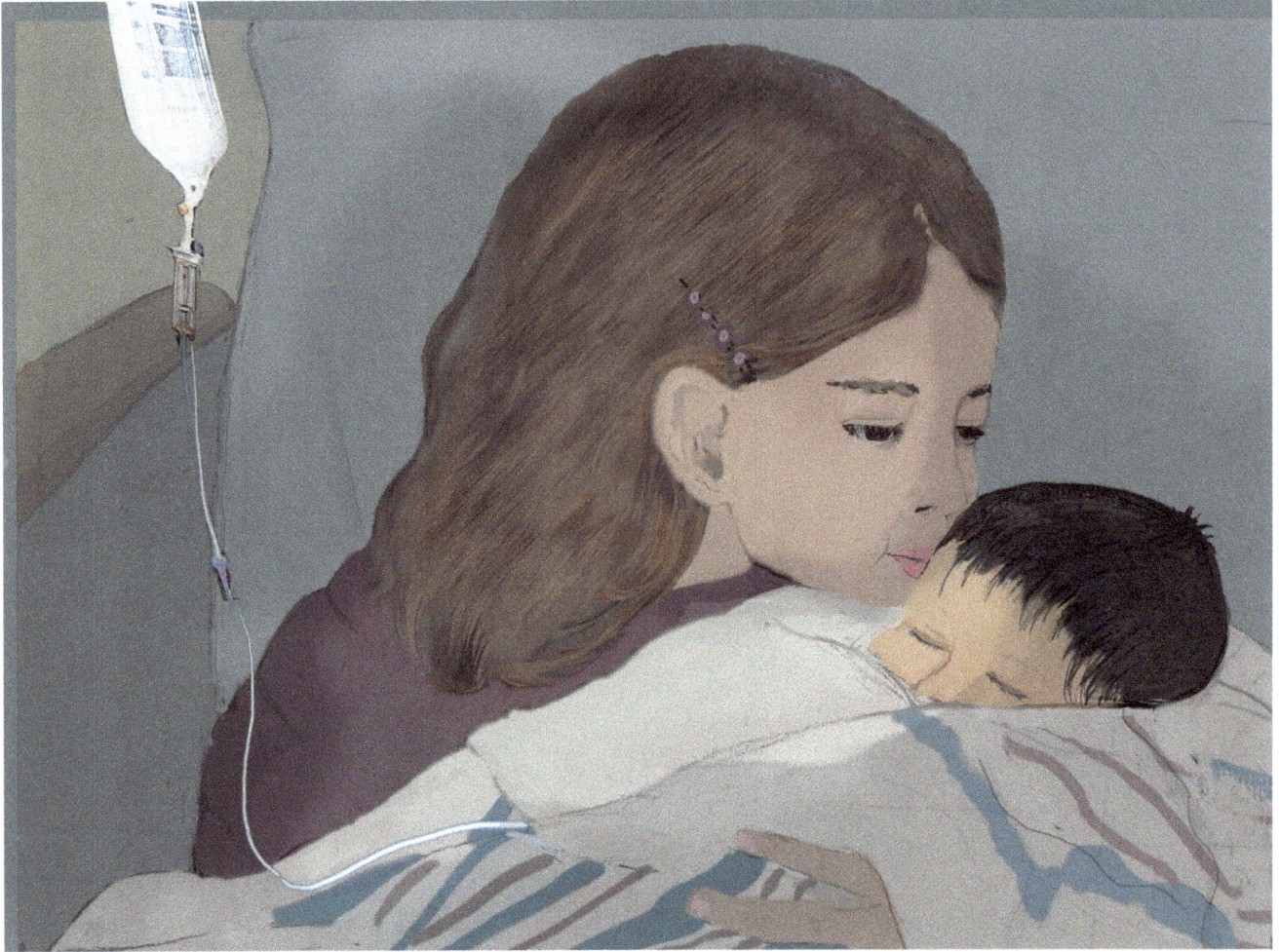

My family and I read a lot about kids with Down syndrome, so we felt ready to meet him.

A day after his birth, Peter got very sick and started throwing up. He could not pass his **meconium**. He was transferred to a bigger hospital at the **NICU**. When I went to see him, I saw that he was attached to many tubes and wires. There were machines making all kinds of beeping sounds all around his hospital crib. I was scared. My parents told me that Peter was doing well, and the machines were there to check his vital signs like his heartbeat and breathing. He also had an **IV** to keep him hydrated.

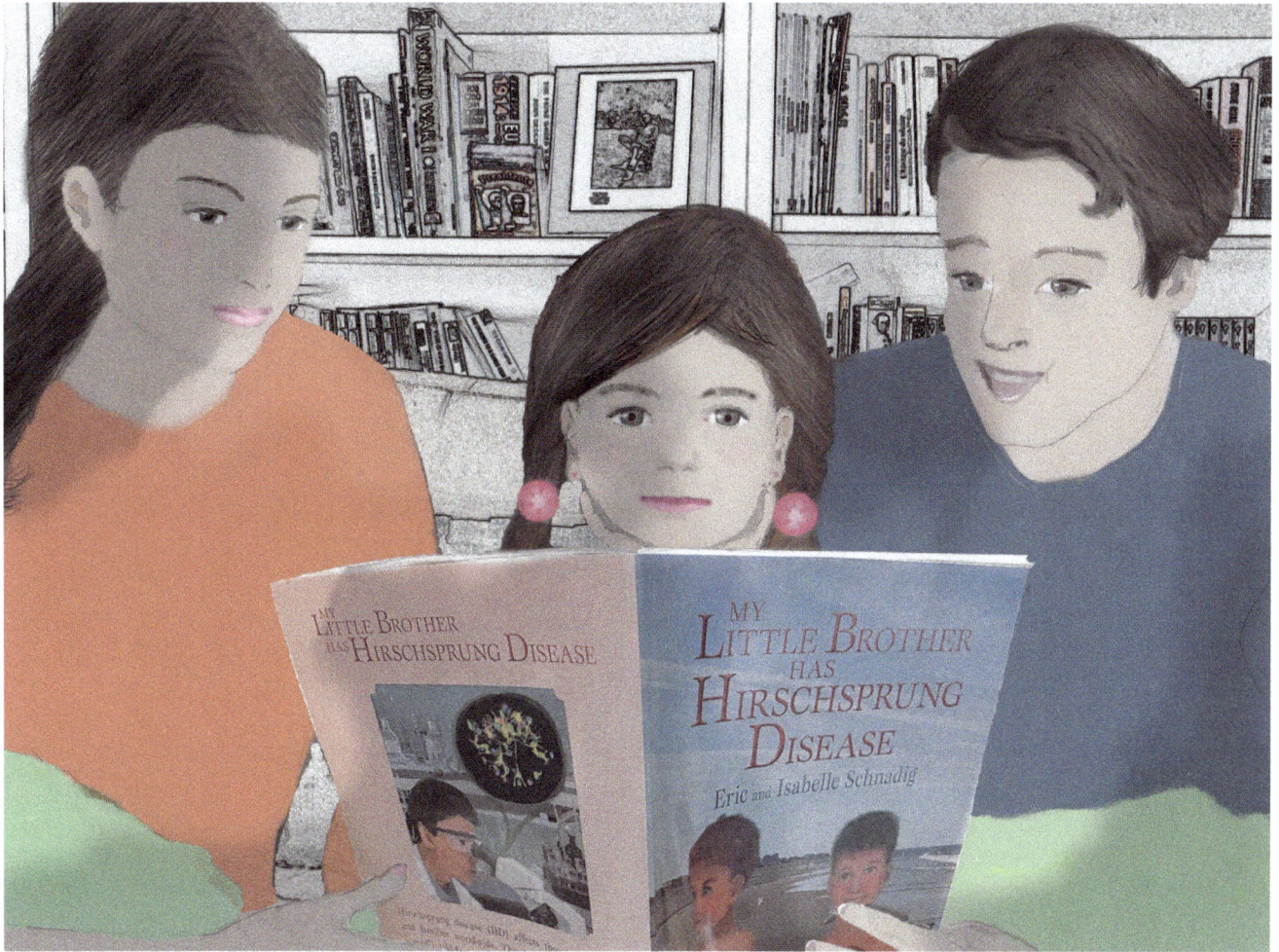

The doctor said Peter needed special tests to find out why he wasn't pooping. They did an **x-ray** of his belly and a **biopsy** of his **rectum**. A few days later, the doctor said Peter had **Hirschsprung Disease**, which is a disease of the **colon**. My baby brother needed surgery to help him poop.

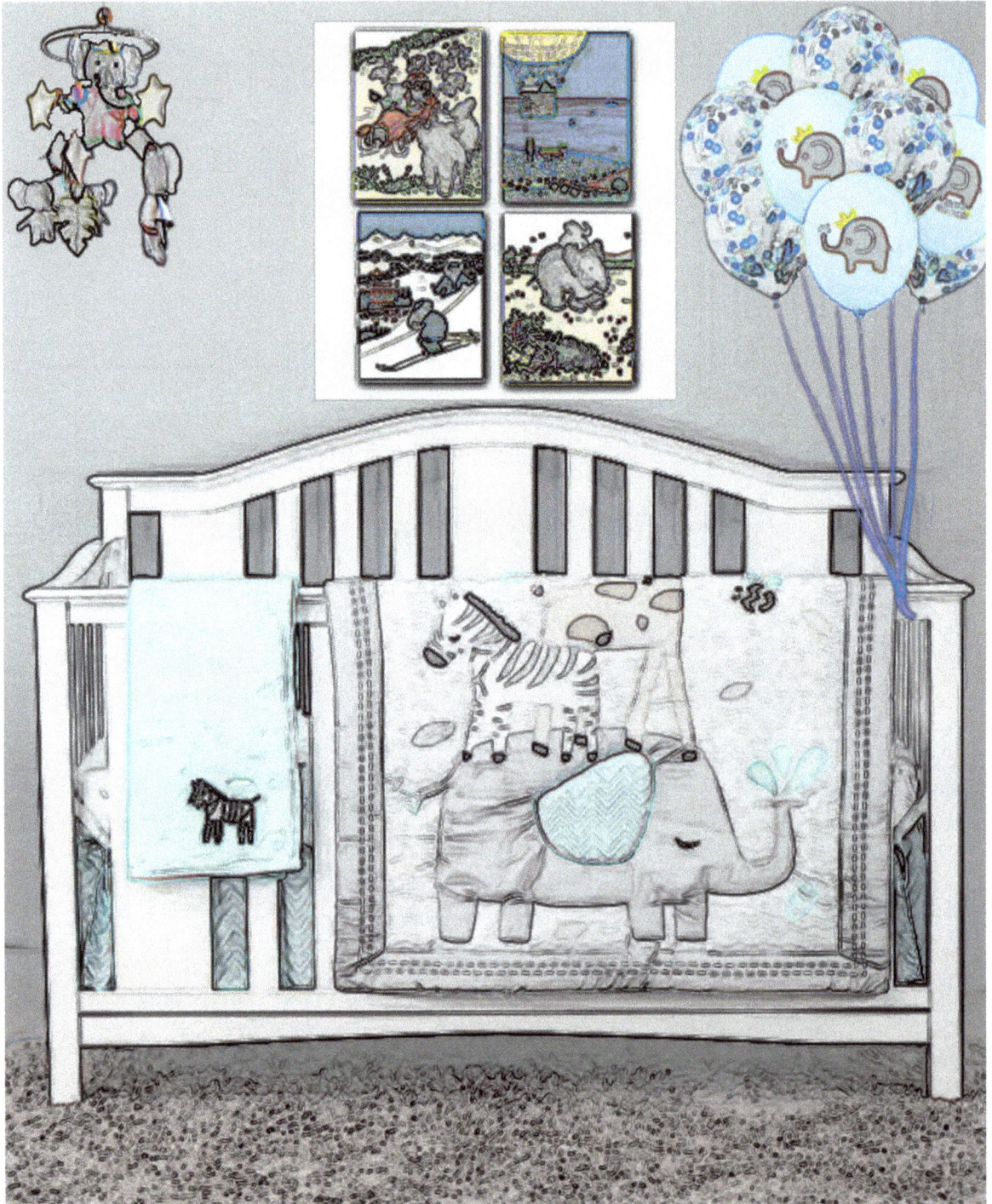

A week after the operation, Peter finally came home. I was so happy that I decorated his whole room to celebrate.

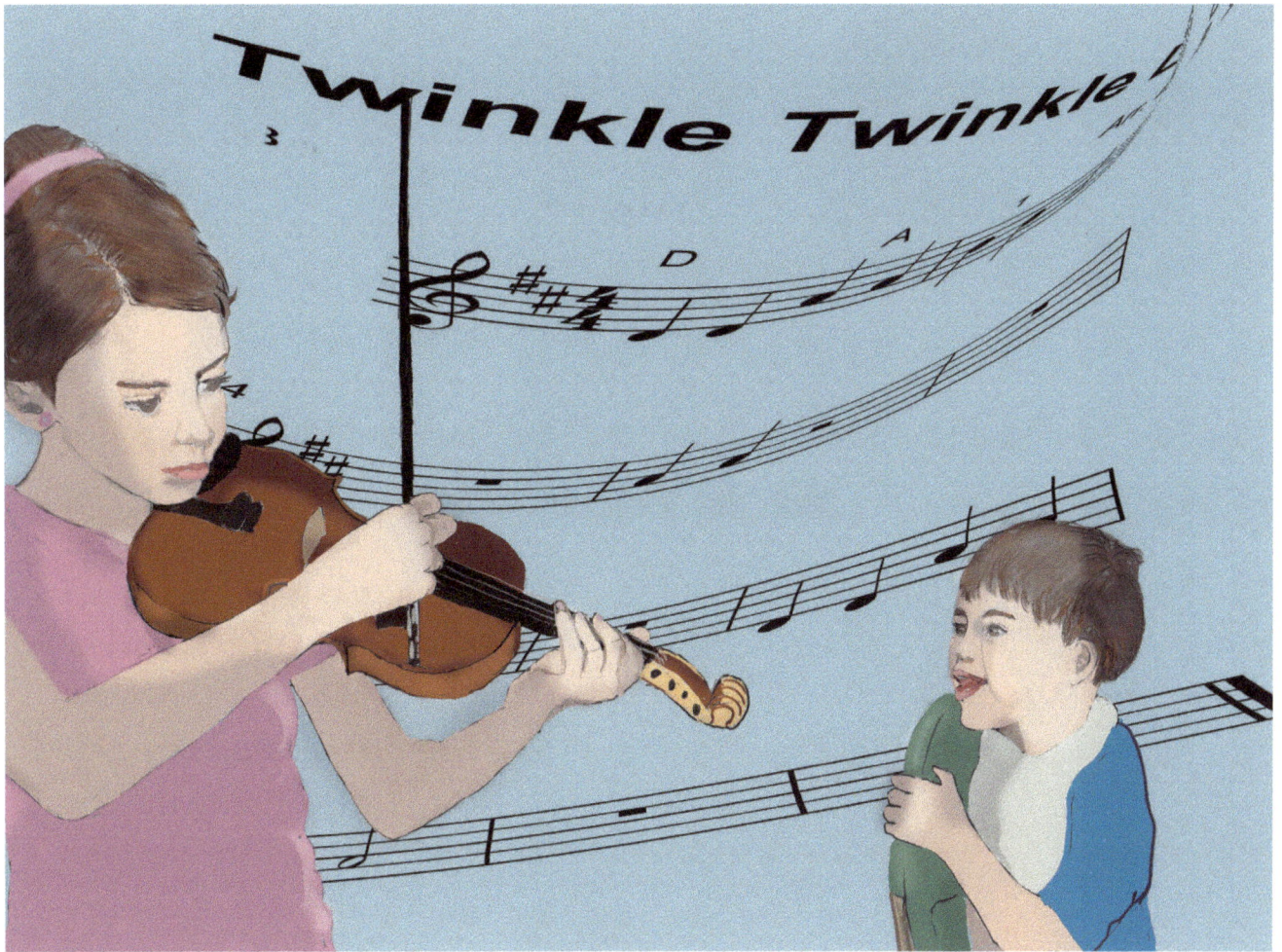

At first, my little brother did not seem too different from my friends' baby siblings. He slept a lot, and when he wasn't sleeping, he was eating or pooping, crying, and smiling. I got to read to him, hold him, and talk to him. I even played the violin because it seemed to soothe him and make him happy.

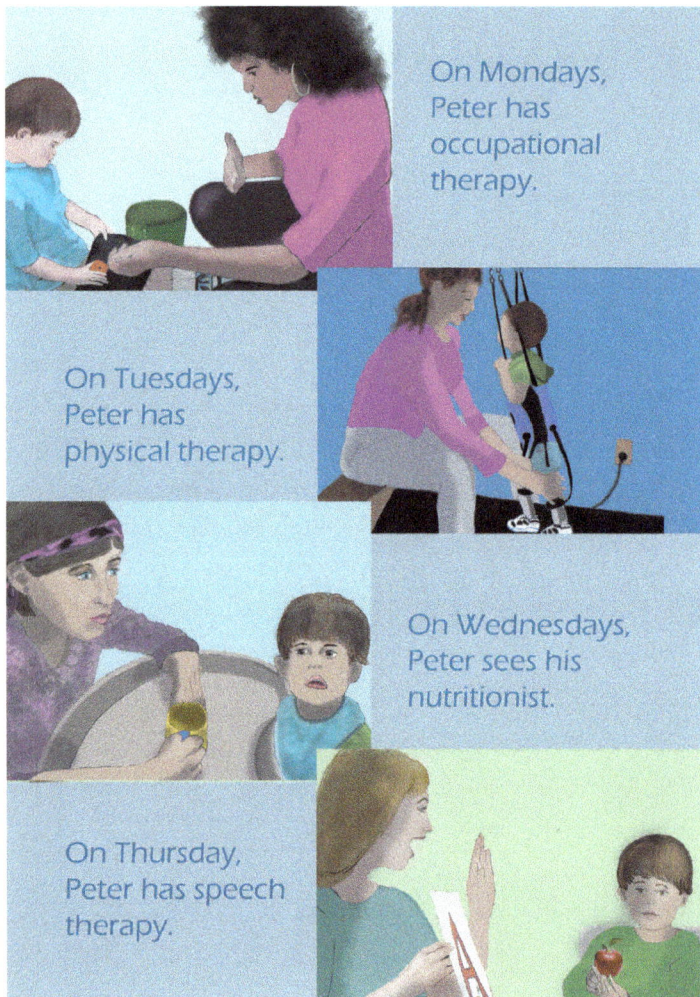

On Mondays, Peter has occupational therapy.

On Tuesdays, Peter has physical therapy.

On Wednesdays, Peter sees his nutritionist.

On Thursday, Peter has speech therapy.

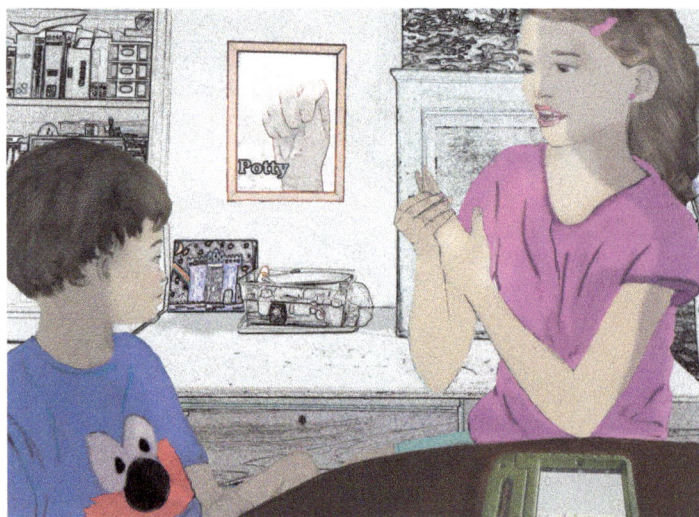

My parents made sure Peter had all the help he needed to stay healthy and flourish. He got a lot of attention from doctors but also from professional **therapists** who came to our house to help him in ways that typical kids didn't need. Peter had his own **occupational therapist**, **physical therapist**, **nutritionist**, and **speech therapist**. Our house was busy all the time! Sometimes I even felt a little jealous of all the attention my brother was getting.

Even though Peter was a toddler, he still could not crawl, stand, or talk. My parents had to carry him everywhere or put him in his stroller. I had to explain this to my friends. I also learned **sign language** so we could speak to each other.

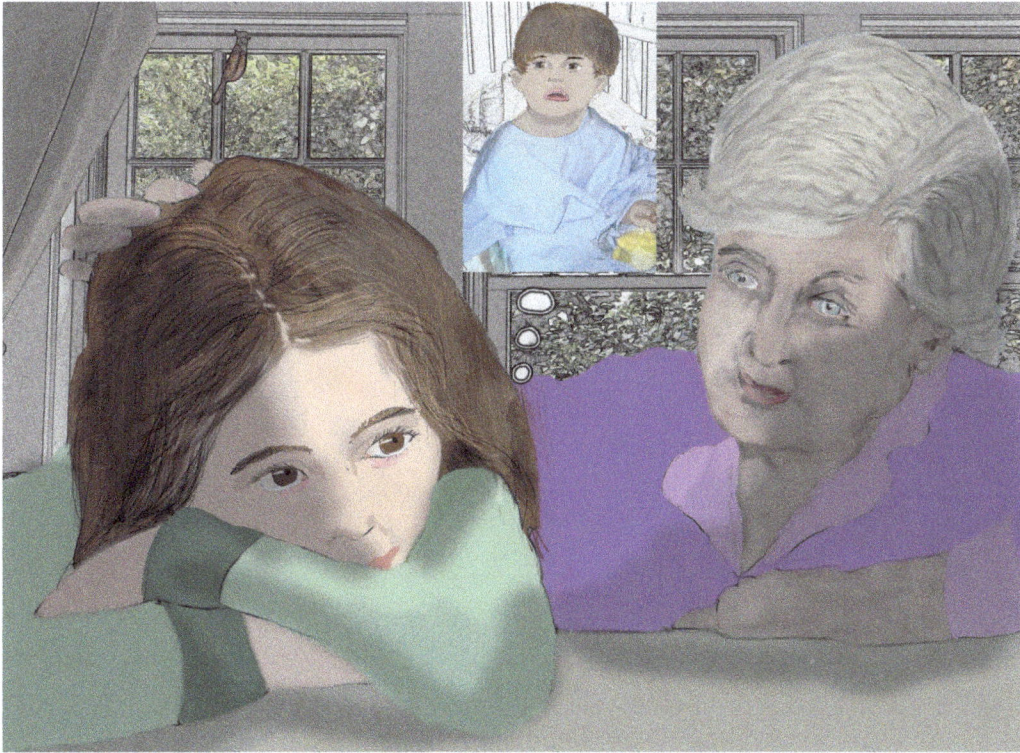

The hardest thing was that Peter started to get sick very often. My parents spent a lot of time at the hospital to make him healthy again. He often just needed some extra hydration to help fight a **virus**, so the doctors usually gave him an IV. We learned to make sure he drank a lot of water to keep him hydrated. One time, he had a terrible **diaper rash** after what my parents called **a Botox treatment** to help him poop. It was a scary week with a lot of diaper changes and having to put Peter in the bath instead of using wipes. His bottom was very sore, and my parents even had to take him to the hospital to treat the diaper rash. During those times, I stayed home with my grandma. I was worried about my little brother but also, I was sad that my life had changed so much. My parents were tired all the time. I used to play boardgames most nights with my parents, but now they were always too tired to play. My friends didn't understand because none of them had a sibling with special needs.

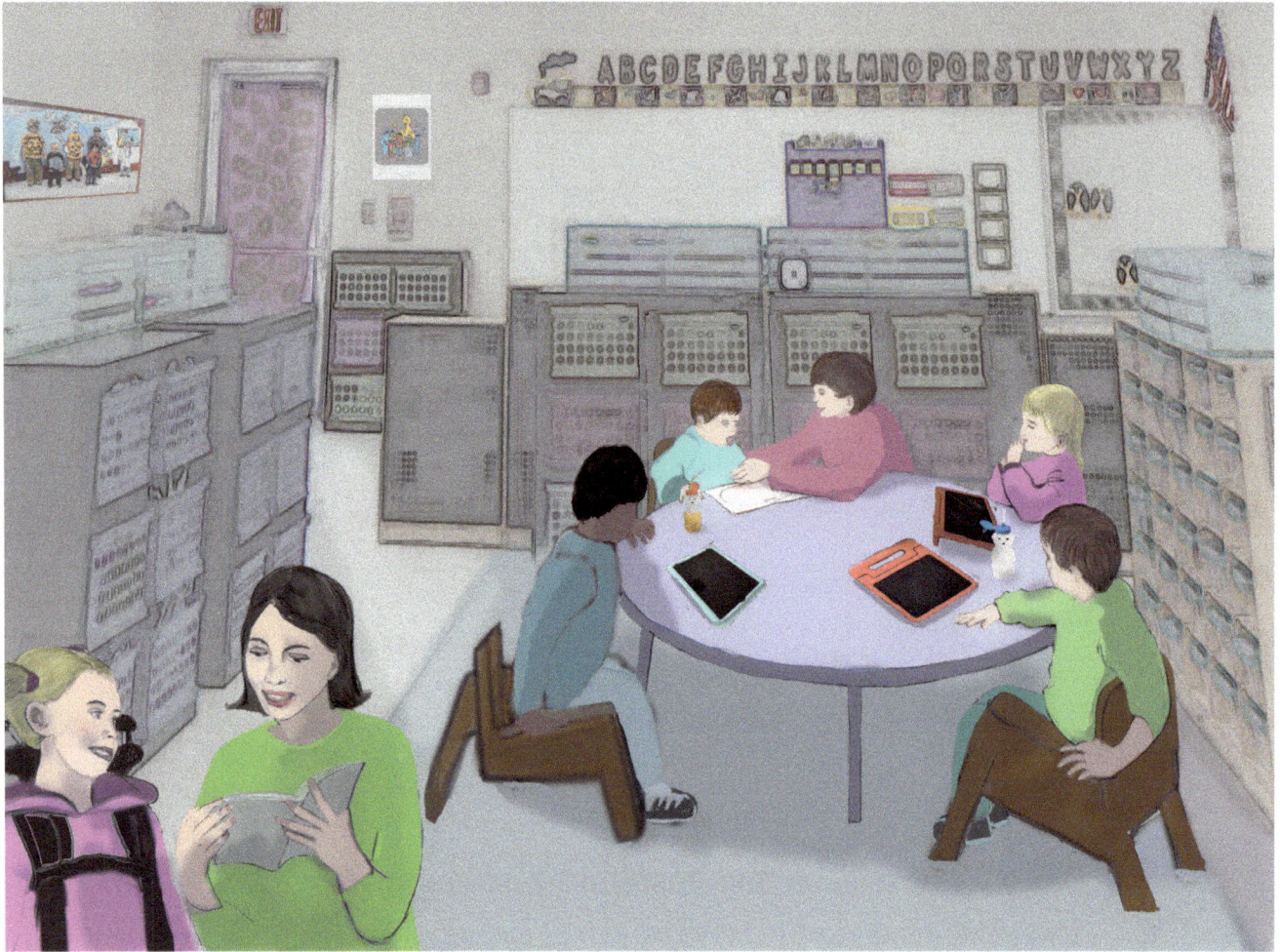

Peter started to get better when he turned five. He didn't have to go to the hospital as often. He was a lot stronger—he could now walk. I was very proud of him. Peter started going to a school that provided **special education** for kids with **special needs**. Even though he still couldn't talk much, he had many great teachers who helped him with everything.

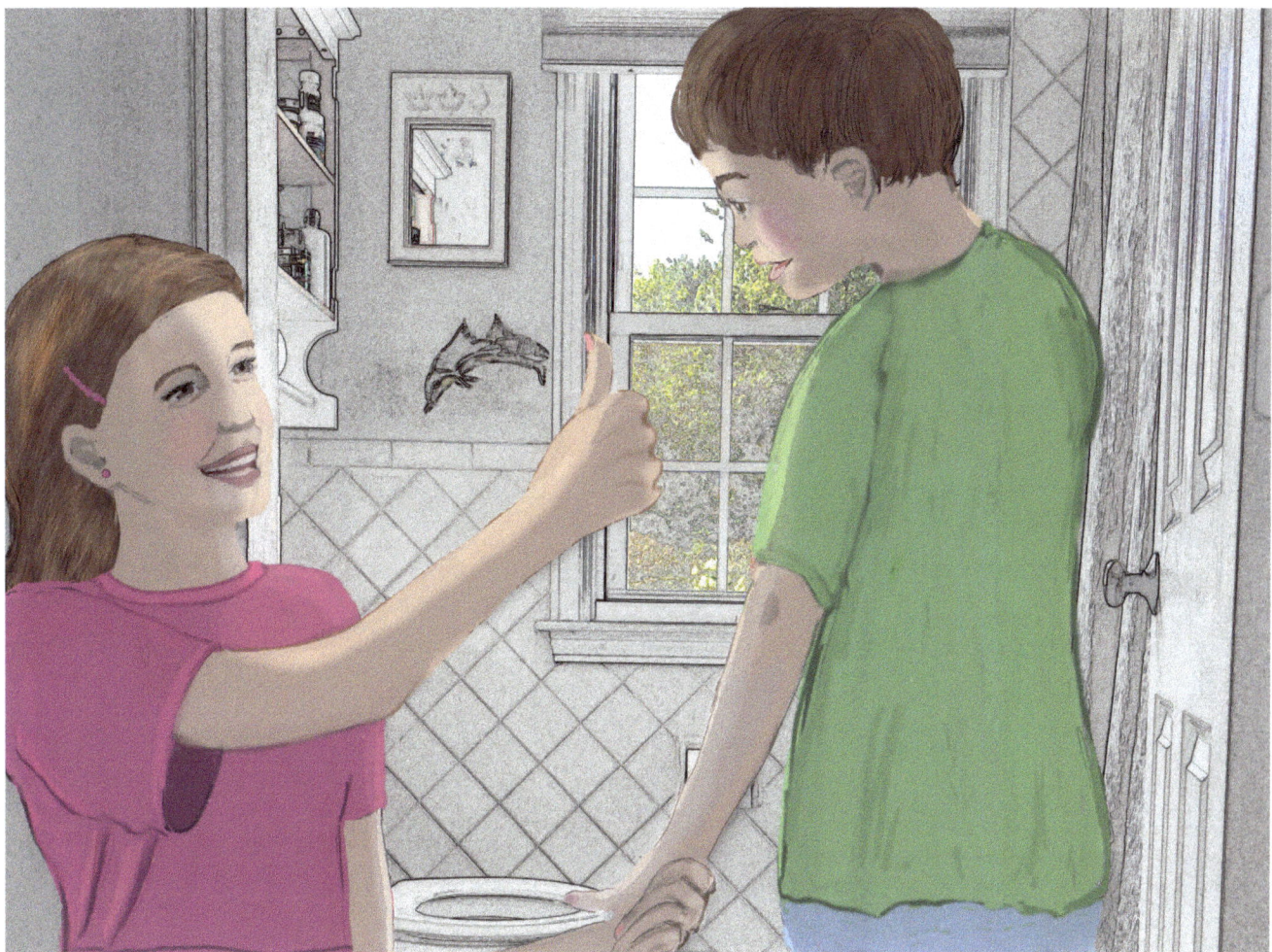

One of the things that did not change over those years was how much my parents talked about Peter and his **bowel movements (BM)**. He still had to wear a diaper because his Hirschsprung Disease caused him to have bathroom accidents. It was always a big deal when he had a BM. We even had a poopy dance to celebrate! When Peter was ten, he finally got toilet trained and wore regular underwear. I was so pleased with him.

I love how my parents always made a big deal for Peter's big and small achievements! Some of the things we celebrated were sitting by himself, crawling, pulling up to stand, walking, speaking more than two words, learning to read, and getting toilet trained. More recently, he learned how to drink with a straw and ask to be excused from dinner to play with his iPad.

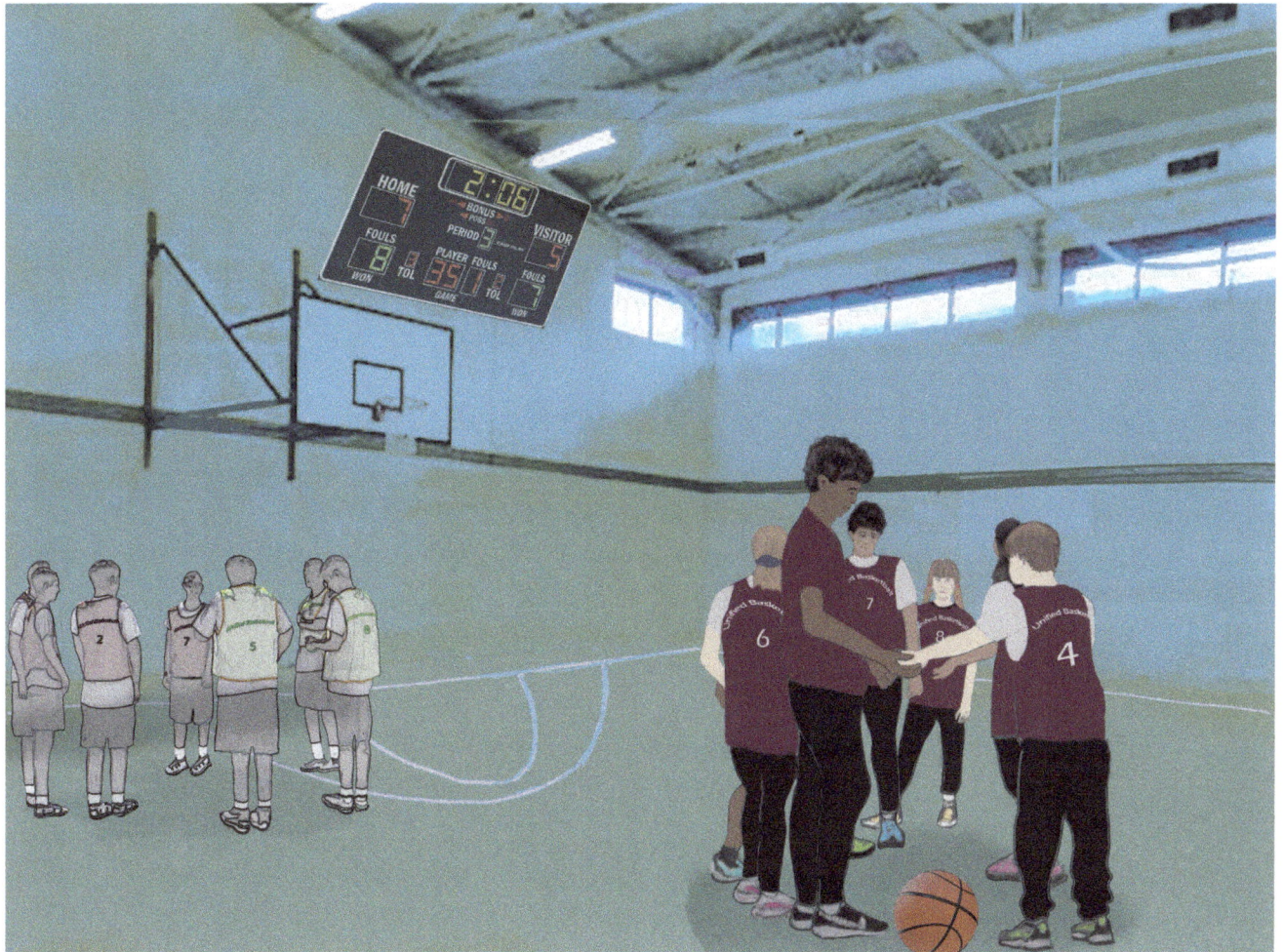

My parents even created some **social stories** to help Peter learn new skills such as drinking from his new cup or getting dressed independently.

Today, my little brother is 16. He is in a special program in my old high school and really loves going to his class every day. He even started doing **Unified Basketball** and **Unified Track**.

Because of his DS, Peter still cannot tell us how he feels when something is wrong or give us information about his day. We do a lot of guessing. And because of his HD, we still have to make sure he drinks enough liquid during the day.

Everything that seems easy for most of us is very challenging for him. That's why my little brother is such a trooper.

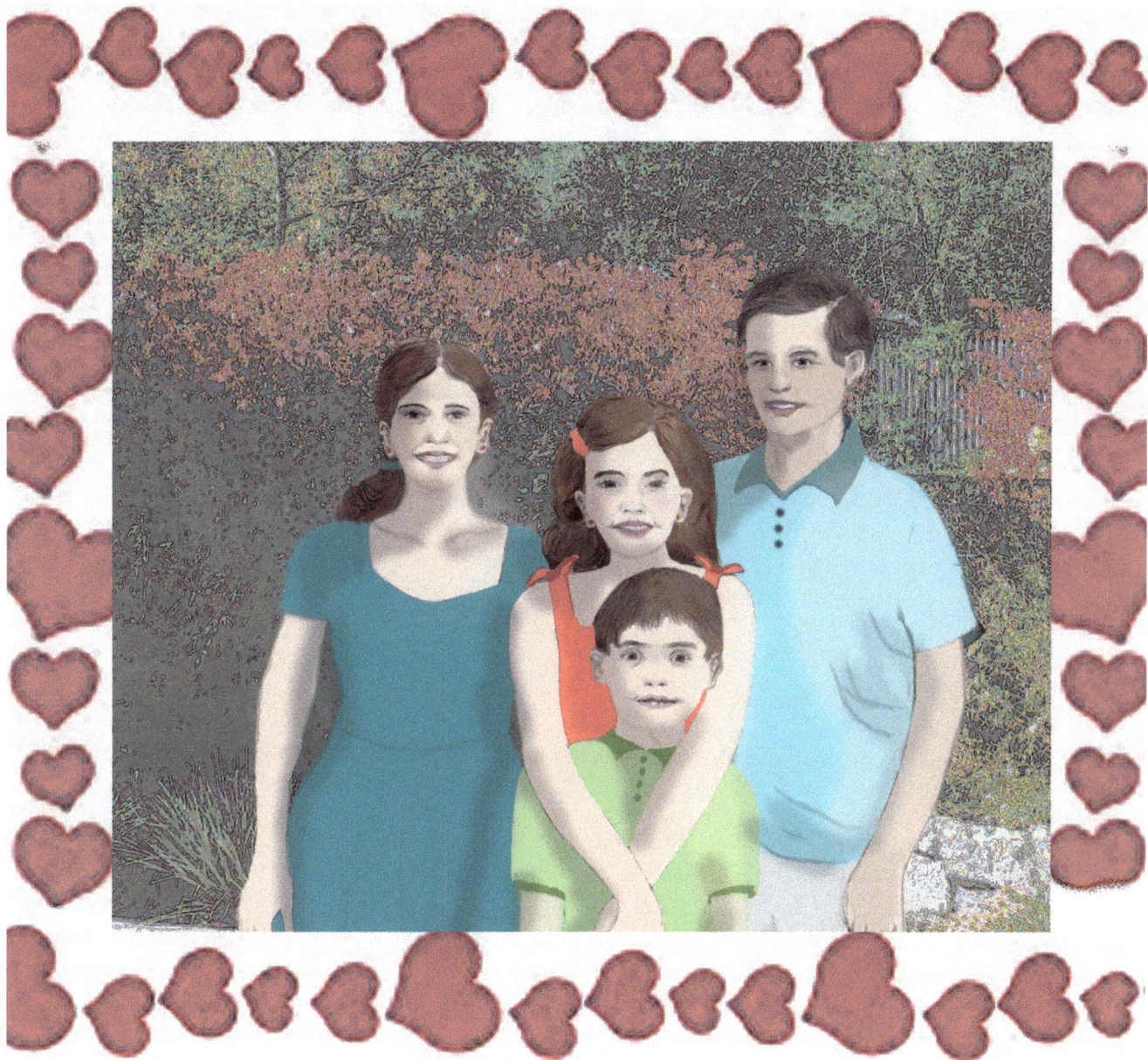

He has two **medical conditions** but still has a smile on his face most of the time. Peter always stays positive and doesn't have a mean bone in his body. He gives me so much love. Peter lives in the moment and is happiest when he is surrounded by friends and family. He has become, at times, the center of our lives but also the ambassador to a world of others struggling with **adversity**.

GLOSSARY

Adversity is a state or instance of serious or continued difficulty or misfortune.

Biopsy is an examination of tissues removed from a living body to discover the presence, cause, or extent of a disease.

Botox treatment is a surgical procedure during which a surgeon injects Botox in the anal sphincter to relieve constipation in children with Hirschsprung Disease.

Bowel movement (BM) is when your body moves waste leftover from digested food through your intestines and out your anus. This process is also known as pooping or defecation.

Chromosomes: To understand why Down syndrome happens, you need to understand a little about chromosomes. What are chromosomes? They're thread-like structures within each cell and are made up of genes. Genes provide the information that decides our traits, from our hair color to whether we're girls or boys. Most people have 23 pairs of chromosomes — half are from your mom and half are from your dad — for a total of 46. But a baby with Down syndrome has an extra chromosome (47 instead of 46), or one chromosome has an extra part. This extra genetic material causes problems with the way their bodies develop.

Colon is the main part of the large intestine that absorbs water and electrolytes from the waste matter. (The parts of the colon are called the ascending, transverse, descending, and sigmoid colon.)

Diaper Rash is redness or irritation that develops on the genitals, buttocks, or thighs. It's the most common skin condition that affects infants, occurring in about half of all babies.

Down Syndrome is a genetic disorder caused when abnormal cell division results in an extra full or partial copy of chromosome 21. There are three types of Down syndrome: Trisomy 21 (95% of cases) is the most common and happens where every cell in the body has three copies of chromosome 21 instead of two; Translocation (4% of cases) in which each cell has part of an extra chromosome 21, or an entirely extra one; Mosaic Down syndrome (1% of cases) where one some cells have an extra chromosome 21. Kids with Down syndrome often have medical problems and trouble learning. But many can go to regular schools, make friends, enjoy life, and get jobs when they're older. Getting special help early — often when they are just babies and toddlers — can be the key to healthier, happier, more independent lives.

Early Childhood Intervention (ECI) is a support and educational system for very young children (aged birth to five) who (in this book) have developmental delays or disabilities.

Hirschsprung Disease is a disease of the large intestine where the nerve cells (also called ganglion cells) are absent, preventing the normal function of the bowel and resulting in the inability to poop normally. Without those cells the colon cannot squeeze and relax, so no poop can come out.

IV is an intravenous (within a vein) therapy. Most often it refers to giving medicine or fluids through a needle or tube inserted into a vein.

Kids with **Special Needs** are children who have been evaluated and determined to have requirements above and beyond what's typical for kids of a similar age and developmental level.

A **Medical Condition** is an illness or a disorder. In the book, it refers to Hirschsprung Disease and Down syndrome.

Meconium is the dark substance forming in the first feces of a newborn infant.

The **NICU** is the neonatal intensive care unit, a special place for sick newborns where they get extra attention from doctors and nurses.

Nutritionist is a person who helps people learn healthy eating habits to improve health and prevent disease. In this book, the person is conducting individual assessments in nutritional history, dietary intake, feeding skills and feeding problems.

Occupational Therapist (OT) is a person who helps a child with special needs improve performance in several areas, such as self-care, school, play, and other activities in which they are required to participate.

Physical Therapist (PT) is a person who works to enhance a child's functional and physical performance in school and other areas of his/her life in which they may face occupational and physical challenges.

Social Story is used to provide guidance and directions for responding to various types of social situations. In this book, the stories are created by the parents to help Peter learn some specific skills, such as getting dressed by himself.

Rectum is the final section of the large intestine, terminating at the anus.

Sign Language is a system of communication using visual gestures and signs, as used by deaf people.

Speech Therapist or **Speech-Language Pathologist (SLP)** is an expert in communication. He/she works with babies up to adults. She/he treats many types of communication and swallowing problems.

Special Education means designed instruction, at no cost to the parents, to meet the unique needs of a child with a disability. Based on the current Individuals with Disabilities Education Act (IDEA), most students with Down syndrome now start in an inclusion classroom, where they are educated alongside neurotypical peers.

Therapist is a person skilled in a particular kind of therapy, such as, in this book, occupational, physical, or speech therapist.

Unified Basketball and **Unified Track** are sports programs in which athletes with and without intellectual disabilities compete together on the same team. It was created by Special Olympics to foster inclusivity and collaboration among people of diverse abilities.

Viruses are tiny particles that cause disease in people, other animals, and plants. Different viruses cause the common cold, influenza, etc.

X-ray is a photographic or digital image of a part of the body.

THE EARLY YEARS WITH YOUR CHILD

During the first five years of Adrien's life, my husband Eric and I had to team up intensively to care for our son. In addition to having HD and DS, Adrien had other significant medical issues, such as vision impairment with glaucoma, severe food and seasonal allergies, and sleep apnea (which is treated with a CPAP mask). There is no doubt that all those medical conditions contributed to all the challenges in Adrien's development, but I do think that HD has probably been the most impactful.

There is no doubt in our minds that those early years of caring for our son have had a negative impact on the attention/care of our three other children during that time. My husband and I were often in a deficit of physical and mental energy. I wish I could have done better at the time. As Adrien grew older, he became more resilient, and our family life became more balanced.

As I reflect on those early years, Adrien's care, and our way of dealing with his medical conditions, I would like to share some of my learnings:

> It is very important to trust your ability to understand your child best. As a parent, you know more about him/her than any other person involved in his/her life. I highly recommend

that you use a calendar to keep track of details such as illness, bowel movements, need for irrigation, introduction to a new food item, etc. It will be so helpful when you try to identify the root cause of a medical issue.

It is also important to acquire knowledge about both conditions and to stay informed about the best therapies.

Above all, take care of yourself. You will require time to recharge your battery, especially in the early years of your child's life. Eric and I were fortunate to be able to afford to hire amazing people to help care for Adrien over all those years. With less resources, I would suggest teaming up with a family in a similar situation to help each other.

Finding a community, such as a support group, will be essential to share your experience with others going through similar challenges.

It is important to take care of your marriage and allow time alone with your partner. When time and energy are scarce, it is easy to drift apart from one another. However, having a strong partnership is so helpful and rewarding as you share the fruits of a full life together.

Make sure to devote regular and one-on-one time with each of your other children.

Your child may never become fully independent. As a result, you will have very important roles to play by being:

- An advocate for him/her. You will remain the person who communicates with educators, doctors, and caregivers.

- A guide for your family members and friends to help them understand, appreciate, and respond to your child/teenager/ adult.

- A decision-maker to help make the best choice for your child during the different stages of his/her life.

I was mostly painting the difficult part of the journey as it is when we need the most help and guidance. I also need to tell you about the easy part of it, when the clouds of the storm have left, and the sun is back. Adrien was a super cute baby and has become a delightful young man; he has more wisdom than anyone I know. He lives fully in the present and loves everyone in his surroundings so deeply and unconditionally. He is also extremely compassionate, emotionally aware, and empathic. In addition, he has a great sense of humor and loves to connect with his friends, peers, and teachers, but also random people. He has the power to make anyone having a bad day smile!

REFERENCES

Beck, Martha. *Expecting Adam: A True Story of Birth, Rebirth, and Everyday Magic*. Harmony/Rodale, 2011.

Bruni, Maryanne. *Fine Motor Skills for Children with Down Syndrome: A Guide for Parents and Professionals*. Woodbine House, 2016.

Couwenhoven, Terri. *The Boys' Guide to Growing Up*. Woodbine House, 2012.

Couwenhoven, Terri. *Teaching Children with Down Syndrome about Their Bodies, Boundaries, and Sexuality: A Guide for Parents and Professionals*. Published by the Woodbine House, 2007.

Friedmacher Florian and **Prem Puri**. *Hirschsprung's disease associated with Down syndrome: a meta-analysis of incidence, functional outcomes, and mortality*. https://pubmed.ncbi.nlm.nih.gov/23943251/

Gill, Barbara. *Changed by a Child: Companion Notes for Parents of a Child with a Disability*. Harmony, 1998.

Kidder, Cynthia, and **Skotko Brian**. *Common Threads: Celebrating Life with Down Syndrome*. Band of Angels Press, 2001.

Klein, Stanley D., and **Kim Schive**, Editors. *You Will Dream New Dreams: Inspiring Personal Stories by Parents of Children with Disabilities*. Kesington Publishing Corp, 2001.

Kumin, Libby. *Early Communication Skills for Children with Down Syndrome; A Guide for Parents and Professionals*. Woodbine House, second edition 2003.

Pueschel, Sigfried M. *A Parent's Guide to Down Syndrome: Toward a Brighter Future.* Brookes Publishing, 2000.

Schnadig, Isabelle and **Eric.** *My Little Brother Has Hirschsprung Disease.* SDP Publishing, 2020.

Simon, Jo Ann. *The Down Syndrome Transition Handbook.* Woodbine House, 2010.

Stein, PsyD, Dr. David. *Supporting Positive Behavior in Children and Teens with Down Syndrome.* Woodbine House, 2016.

Stray-Gundersen, Karen. *Babies with Down Syndrome: A New Parent's Guide.* Woodbine House, 1995.

Stuve-Bodeen, Stephanie, Pam and **Devito.** *We'll Paint the Octopus Red.* Woodbine House, 1998.

Mattheis, Philip, and **Susan Eberly.** *Medical & Surgical Care for Children with Down Syndrome: A Guide for Parents.* Woodbine House, 1995.

Winders, Patricia C. *Gross Motor Skills in Children with Down Syndrome: A Guide for Parents and Professionals.* Woodbine House, Inc. 1997.

Zuckoff, Mitchel. *Choosing Niai: A Family's Journey.* Beacon Press, 2002.

Resources

A Family Guide to Transition Services in Massachusetts. Published by the Massachusetts Rehabilitation Commission in Collaboration with the Federation for Children with Special Needs. 2013

Family TIES of Massachusetts. Parent-to-parent information and support network for families of children with special needs. *Massachusetts Family TIES (massfamilyties.org)*

Down Syndrome Clinic to You or DSC2U. http:www.dsc2u.org

Massachusetts Down Syndrome Congress (mdsc). https://mdsc.org

National Down Syndrome Congress. https://www.ndsccenter.org. Email: *info@ndscenter.org*

"Founded in 1973, we are the leading national resource of support and information for anyone touched by or seeking to learn about Down syndrome, from the moment of prenatal diagnosis through adulthood. The NDSC offers programs for families and professionals, and we're always looking for new ways to support individuals with Down syndrome. We provide resources on a wide array of topics, some that we've created at our center and others that we share from trusted sources. If you are looking for something specific and don't readily find it on our site, want to dig deeper into a topic, or just need someone to listen, please call the center at 1-800-232-NDSC (6372) Monday through Friday from 9 a.m. to 5:30 p.m. eastern time. We are here to help!" Also they have a list of Down Syndrome Clinic by state: *Down Syndrome Clinic Listing | National Down Syndrome Congress (ndsccenter.org)*

National Down Syndrome Society (NDSS). www.ndss.org. Email: *info@ndss.org.* NDSS empowers individuals with Down syndrome and their families by driving policy change, providing resources, engaging with local communities, and shifting public perceptions.

A Family Guide to Transition Services in Massachusetts. Published by the Massachusetts Rehabilitation Commission in Collaboration with the Federation for Children with Special Needs. 2013

National Down Syndrome Society. National Down Syndrome Society (NDSS) NDSS empowers individuals with Down syndrome and their families by driving policy change, providing resources, engaging with local communities, and shifting public perceptions.

About the Author

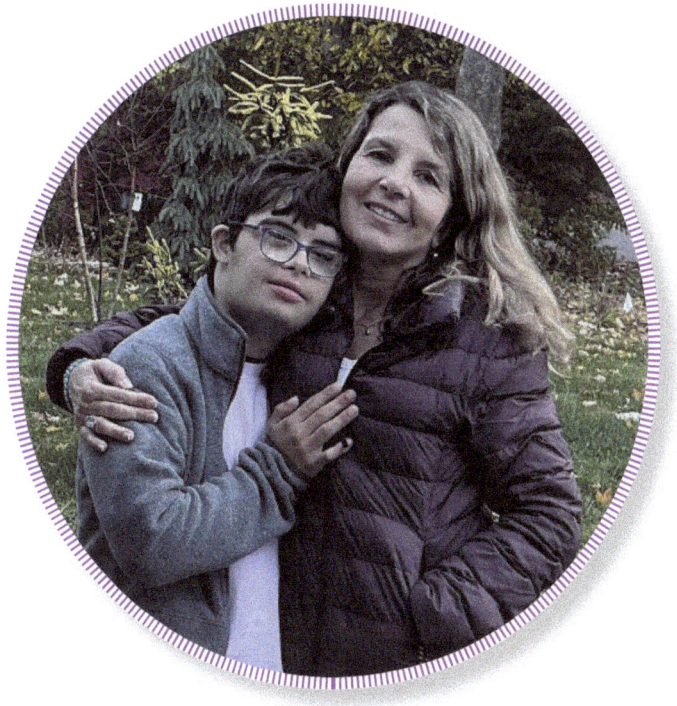

Isabelle Schnadig is a French-American artist and illustrator, and author of children's books on difficult subjects such as the Hirschsprung and Alzheimer's diseases. She lives in Concord, MA, with her husband and her younger son. She is also the co-founder of Reachirschsprung (*www.reachhd.org*), the foundation which provides research, education and advocacy for children and families with Hirschsprung disease. Her new book is designed to help the children and their family that have a dual diagnosis: Down syndrome and Hirschsprung.

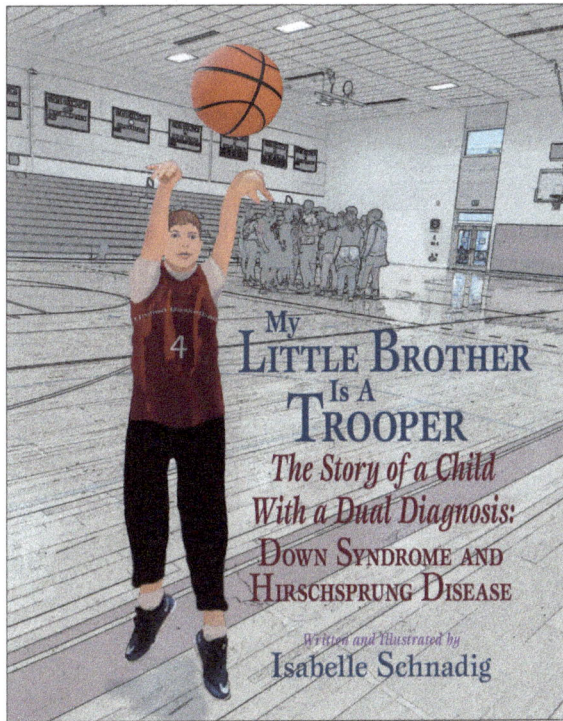

My Little Brother Is a Trooper
Isabelle Schnadig

www.reachhd.org

Also available in ebook format

Available at all major bookstores

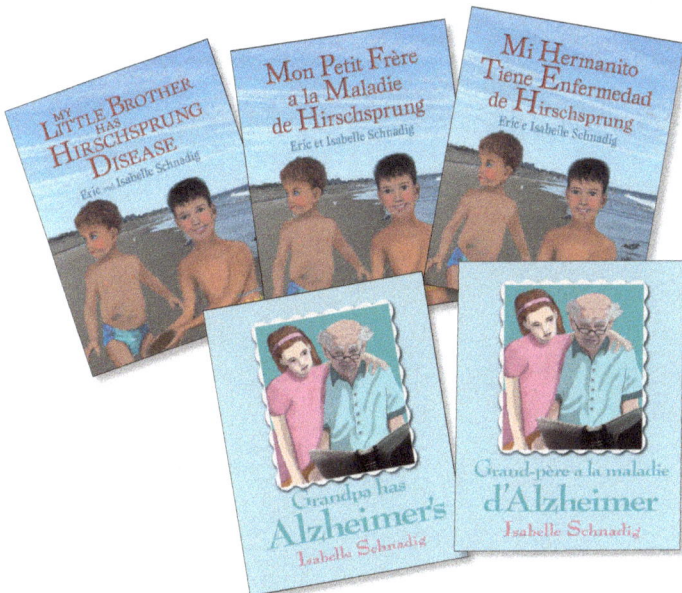

Other books by Eric and Isabelle Schnadig:

My Little Brother Has Hirschsprung Disease
Mon Petit Frère a la Maladie de Hirschsprung
Mi Hermanito Tiene Enfermedad
Grandpa has Alzheimer's
Grand-père a la Maladie d'Alzheimer

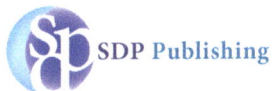

SDP Publishing

www.SDPPublishing.com
Contact us at: info@SDPPublishing.com